# GLUTEN-FREE
# 5-INGREDIENT
# COOKBOOK

40 Easy Recipes with 30 Minutes or Less Prep Time for a Healthy New You!

**GRETCHEN FREEMAN**

# Copyright © 2020



# LEGAL & DISCLAIMER

# TABLE OF CONTENTS

# GLUTEN-FREE DIET

## What is gluten-free diet?

These are meals prepared by taking out foodstuffs that contain the gluten protein from food. Gluten belongs to a class of proteins present in foods like wheat, rye, and barley. The name gluten is derived from the word "glue" (a Latin word). This protein produces a sticky effect in food, most especially in flours.

This sticky property aids to form a gluey network that enables certain foods to swell during preparation. It also produces an elastic texture in those food. Sometime, these proteins can be difficult for people to digest, and are thought to aggravate or even cause some health issues. A meal with zero gluten can provide many health benefits, particularly for individuals with digestive issues due to the celiac disease. Foods having no gluten content can help improve such digestive symptoms, minimize inflammation, release vitality and stimulate weight loss.

## Why gluten-free cooking?

Some people need to avoid gluten to save their lives, while others simply feel better and believe they are healthier without it. Some gluten-intolerant people become uncomfortable after consuming gluten-rich foods.

People with extreme sensitivity are usually referred to as having a celiac disease. This disease is a condition in which the body harms itself by mistake and it affects more than one percent of the population. Celiac disease can cause great harm in the body, most especially in the intestines. There is another condition called "gluten sensitivity" that also causes problems with gluten. Many foods are made with gluten-containing ingredients. So it's important that those who are intolerant to gluten avoid it completely. If not, you will experience severe discomfort and adverse health effects. When buying your products, check ingredient labels closely.

Gluten-free meals are becoming more popular in the US, with more grocery stores carrying gluten-free products and more restaurants adapting to gluten-free requests than ever before. It's estimated that 30% of all Americans avoid gluten, but only a small percentage of these have celiac illness or a severe gluten allergy.

## Healthy foods with zero gluten

Luckily, there is a wide range of substitute food that can replace gluten-free products in the market. With these substitutes, you can switch from gluten-based foods to gluten-free meals more easily without forfeiting essential nutrients.

There are some modified gluten-free products such as gluten-free breakfast cereals, pasta, bread, sweet cookies and so on. The food section of most supermarkets and other specialized stores usually have stock of various gluten-free foods. There are several other delicious alternative meals that you can enjoy and also provide you with sufficient nutrients. The foods listed below are gluten-free and natural without any modification:

- **Fish and Meats**. Most fish and meats, except processed meats are gluten-free.

- **Eggs**. All eggs are free of gluten.

- **Dairy**. Natural dairy products like cow's milk and fresh yogurt are void of gluten. On the other hand, processed dairy products are likely to contain gluten, which is why it is important to read food labels.

- **Vegetables and Fruits**. All vegetables and fruits are gluten-free.

- **Grains**. These include cereals like rice, sorghum, sweet corn, buckwheat, millet, tapioca, and other underutilized grains. (Check the food labels.)

- **Seeds/Nuts.** No gluten protein in seeds and nuts.

- **Margarine/oils.** No gluten protein in butter and vegetable oils.

- **Herbs/spices.** No gluten protein in most spices and herbs.

- **Food beverages**. No gluten protein in most beverages. Nonetheless, if you're not certain if a particular food item has gluten or not, it's imperative that you review the labels before making your purchase.

## Alternative ingredients for grains

Most of the grains available naturally have gluten. Nevertheless, we still have other nutritious gluten-free cereals available for consumption too. These grains do not only serve as alternatives for grains such as barley, wheat or rye, these gluten-free cereals also provide exceptional features:

- **Wheat flour:** You can substitute wheat flour with flour produced from corn, soy or rice. There are also baking powder products with zero gluten available in the market.

- NOTE: Baking with gluten-free flour may turn out to be a little drier, and the dough may not rise like the normal flour. It may also feel like it has a crumbly texture to the hand.

- **Breadcrumbs:** It can be replaced with crumbled wheat-free crackers, shredded parmesan especially when preparing chicken nuggets, meat loaf, deep fried chicken and so on.

- **Arrowroot:** has more fiber than cornstarch. Although its texture, appearance, and gluten-free properties resemble that of cornstarch, arrowroot has the ability to thicken up a liquid more easily than cornstarch. Therefore, arrowroot is a great alternative to cornstarch.

- **Millet**: Actually a grass — with a small seed that grows in a variety of shapes, sizes, and colors.

- **Montina**: Montina is actually a trademarked name by a company called Amazing Grains. Montina is a type of flour made from Indian rice grass.

- **Buckwheat**: Buckwheat is a type of fruit plant. It is also called kasha.

- **Job's tears**: A tropical plant that produces gluten-free grains, it is usually processed and cooked just like normal grain food.

## What foods to avoid?

Below are kinds of food containing gluten that celiac patients should avoid. Although at first, a gluten-free meal can seem terribly restrictive, it's actually not that hard to follow once you get used to it. A celiac patient that follows a well-balanced gluten-free food is expected to lead a healthy life!

Check out the list:

- Most foods containing wheat flours, oats, barley

- Pastry

- Wheat starch

- Mayonnaise, sauces, sweet marinades, soy sauce

- Malt flavoring and vinegar (major ingredients in most breakfast cereals)

- Canned meat or fish

- Most natural flavoring

- Grain-based beer or spirits

Gluten can also be found in other foods such as confectioneries, sausages, sauces, dressings and other condiments.

## How to Check for Gluten Ingredients on Food Labels.

Knowing how to read a food label is the key to happily staying gluten-free. Here's what you need to know. Food labels come in all shapes and sizes. Some are clear, easy to read, and provide all the information you need. Others are confusing, and leave you with more questions than they answer.

When you follow a gluten-free diet, the most important part of a food label is the ingredients list usually found on the back or side of the package. In the ingredients list, food producers must accurately list the ingredients found in a food. So this is the part you will want to read first. But don't look for the word "gluten." Instead look for these words: wheat, rye, barley or malt. Oats on most labels are also off limits. The exception is "specialty" gluten-free oats in a food labeled gluten-free.

The Food Allergen Labeling and Consumer Protection Act (FALCPA) guarantees that if a food contains wheat in any form, you will read the word "wheat" on the label. It also means you no longer have to worry about ingredients like modified food starch or hydrolyzed vegetable protein. If any ingredient is made from wheat, the label will tell you.

Be aware, but not alarmed, that FALCPA covers foods regulated by the Food and Drug Administration (FDA). This includes all packaged food except meat, eggs and poultry, which are regulated by the U.S. Department of Agriculture (USDA). You can feel a high level of confidence that these items, which are naturally gluten-free when plain, are as well labeled as those regulated by the FDA.

Rye and barley are not covered by FALCPA. But rye is rarely, if ever, used in a food in a form other than flour or grain and would always appear in the ingredients list.

Another way to raise your confidence level is to promise yourself that you will read the label every time you purchase a product, regardless of how many times you have previously read the same label and found the item safe. The dirty secret is that things can change – and they do, often enough to make this promise important. It's a bit like buckling your seat belt each time you get behind the wheel, despite never having needed it previously. You just never know what might happen.

# 40 GLUTEN-FREE RECIPES

**NOTE**: In each of the recipes described below, salt, pepper, sugar, oil, and water are not included among the five ingredients.

Also note that the following ingredients used in the recipes are gluten-free versions. They include flour, oats, dough, bread, broths, pastry, tortillas and egg roll wrappers.

# BREAKFAST

## 1. Blueberry Pie Overnight Oats

Preparation time - 20 minutes

**Ingredients**

- 1 cup old fashioned oats

- 1 cup unsweetened vanilla almond milk

- 1 medium bowl of blueberry Greek yogurt

- 1 handful fresh blueberries

- 1 tbsp granola

**Instructions**

1. Mix the oats and almond milk in a container and allow to sit overnight.

2. In the morning, layer the oats, blueberry Greek yogurt and fresh berries.

3. Top with the granola!

# 2. Lemon Overnight Oats

Preparation time - 5 minutes

## Ingredients

- ¾ cup dairy-free milk

- juice of ½ a lemon

- 1 tsp maple syrup

- ¾ cup rolled oats

- 1 tbsp chia seeds

## Instructions

1. Combine all ingredients in a jar/bowl, add a little salt and cover with lid.

2. Keep in fridge overnight and enjoy the next morning.

# 3. Gluten-free Chocolate Chia Pudding

Preparation time - 15 minutes

## Ingredients

- 1 cup non-dairy milk (coconut or almond milk)

- 1 ½ tbsp raw cacao powder

- 2 ½ tbsp chia seeds

- 3 Medjool dates, pitted

## Instructions

1. Mix the entire ingredients in a blender and blend until you have a smooth pudding mixture and everything has combined properly.

2. Transfer the mixture into a bowl and cover it.

3. Keep in the fridge for 2 hours, or overnight.

4. Share the mixture into 2 mason jars.

Toppings: garnish with fresh pineapple, chia seeds, coconut milk, cacao nibs, or gluten-free granola.

## 4. Sweet Potato Hash Sausage and Roasted Poblano Pepper

Preparation time - 20 minutes

**Ingredients**

- 1 ½ lb Italian chicken sausage

- 2 ½ tbsp melted coconut oil

- 1 big poblano pepper

- 5 eggs

- 2 lbs sweet potatoes, diced

- salt and pepper to taste

**Instructions**

1. Pre-heat the oven till it reaches 400° F.

2. Rub coconut oil on the sweet potatoes, and a little pepper and salt.

3. Spread foil on baking sheet and serve sweet potatoes on it along with the poblano.

4. Allow to grill for 6 minutes, then mix by tossing and cook for another 3 minutes.

5. Extract the poblano pepper into a bowl and cover up.

6. Grill the sweet potatoes for another 4 minutes. As the potatoes are grilling, roast sausage in another pan.

7. Add the sausage to the potatoes and roast for one minute.

8. Remove the skin of the poblano pepper, cut out the seeds, then dice.

9. Mix the sausage, poblano pepper and sweet potatoes together.

10. Make 4 craters in the mixture and whisk in the eggs in each crater. Cover and cook for 12 minutes.

11. Alternatively, you can boil the eggs for 4 - 6 minutes and pour into the mixture.

12. Serve and enjoy.

# 5. Gluten-Free Dog Treats

Preparation time - 15 min

## Ingredients

- 1 cup peanut butter or nut butter of choice

- 1 ½ cups puree (potato or pumpkin puree)

- 2 cups coconut flour

- 5 large eggs

- 1 cup coconut oil

## Instructions

1. Heat up the grill to about 400° F.

2. Add the entire ingredients to form a dough in a large bowl, then mold to form a ball.

3. Spread the dough on a doubled parchment paper, then place your cookie cutters to shape the dough. Lift the cutter to reveal a shaped cookie.

4. Transfer to a lined baking sheet.

5. Bake the cookies in the oven for about 15 minutes or till the cookies are hard enough.

6. Allow the cookies to cool down.

# 6. Egg Muffins with Cauliflower Rice and Ham

Preparation time - 15 minutes

## Ingredients

- 3 large eggs

- 1 cup spinach (lightly packed), chopped into bite-sized pieces

- 1 cup cauliflower, chopped into bite-sized pieces

- ¾ cup of ham (heavily packed), diced into bite-sized cubes

- salt and pepper to taste

## Instructions

1. Warm up your oven to 300° F and prepare the muffin tin with sufficient cooking spray. Keep to one side.

2. In a processor, grind the cauliflower carefully till it looks grainy like rice. Keep to one side.

3. Using a big bowl, whisk the eggs thoroughly then mix together with the rest of the ingredients. Add seasoning, salt and pepper as desired. Combine thoroughly.

4. Divide the final combination into 6 muffin tins and bake for 15 minutes.

5. Allow the muffins to cool before serving. ENJOY.

# 7. Breakfast Skillet

Preparation time – 20 minutes

## Ingredients

- ¾ - 1 lb organic ground turkey (or grass-fed beef)

- 1 cup salsa, as desired

- 6 organic eggs

## Instructions

1. Heat skillet with oil over medium heat, and place turkey into it. Cook until turkey browns and no pink remains.

2. Add in salsa and mix to combine, then let it cook together for 2-3 minutes.

3. Crack in eggs and cover skillet for 7 minutes or till the egg whites becomes opaque.

# 8. Gluten-free Shrimp Jicama Tacos

Preparation time - 10 min

## Ingredients

- 1 ½ jicama, peeled and cut into taco-shell sizes

- ¾ cup pineapple

- Marinara sauce or your choice of sauce

- 5 big shrimp, cooked and diced

- ¾ tsp seasoning (Pico Piquin)

## Instructions

1. Mix the entire ingredients except sauce and jicama. Allow the new combination to marry for five minutes.

2. Set out the jicama taco shells and share mixture among the jicama. Drizzle it with your sauce and serve with additional Pico Piquin!

# LUNCH

## 9. Turkey and Cavolo Nero Cabbage Meatballs

Preparation time – 15 minutes

### Ingredients

- 14 oz turkey mince (I used breast meat because it's all I could get, but thigh would be good too)

- 1 garlic clove, peeled and chopped

- 3 cavolo nero leaves, the central tough stalk removed and the leaves chopped fairly finely

- 1 tbsp coconut oil, for frying

- a pinch of salt to taste

### Instructions

1. Empty the packet of mince into a mixing bowl. Add the chopped garlic, the chopped cavolo nero leaves, and the pinch of salt and mix well, but don't over-mix.
2. Heat one tablespoon oil in a largish frying pan and, forming the mince mixture into small meatballs, drop them gently into the pan. You might need to do this in batches, if you have a smaller pan - don't overcrowd them or you might find that they steam cook rather than fry and turn golden.
3. I brown the meatballs, turning them on all sides and cooking for around 5 minutes and then finish them off in the oven, at gas mark 6/400°F for another 10 minutes, until fully cooked through.

This way, you've got the hob free for your veggies or side dishes that you're going to serve them with. We love to serve them with spiralized courgette/zucchini.

4. They're also lovely hot or cold - keep a batch in the fridge and take them out on a picnic when the weather gets warmer.

# 10. Easy Lemon Basil Zoodles

Preparation time – 10 minutes

## Ingredients

- 1 medium-large zucchini, spiralized

- 1 clove of garlic, minced

- 2 - 3 tbsp of olive oil

- salt and pepper to taste

- shredded basil

- lemon wedges (optional)

## Instructions

1. Prepare zoodles and mince garlic, then heat olive oil in large pan over medium to low heat.

2. Add in garlic and fresh shredded basil. Cook for approximately a minute or so.

3. Add in zoodles and sauté along with the basil and garlic. Season with salt and pepper to taste. Cook zoodles for about 3-5 minutes, tossing frequently until al dente.

4. Remove from heat and spoon onto the plate. Garnish with basil and lemon wedges, if desired.

5. Serve and enjoy!

# 11. Healthy Turkey Meatballs with Italian Herbs

Preparation time - 15 min

## Ingredients

- 1 lb ground turkey (organic)

- 2 tsp Italian herb blend

- 2 tsp black pepper

- ¾ tsp oregano

- salt to taste

Optional

- 1 tsp parsley

- 1 tsp garlic powder

## Instructions

Incorporating the herbs into the turkey.

1. Mix herb blend in a small ramekin.

2. In a medium bowl, add herb blend, salt, black pepper, oregano, and optional ingredients to ground turkey in portions. Do not over-mix. The ingredients should be incorporated and mixed through, but not overworked.

3. Form golf ball sized meatballs, then place on plate. Cover meatball plate with plastic wrap and let sit for 10 minutes at least to allow to meld.

Cooking the meatballs.

1.  Turn oven to 350° F. Line a cookie sheet or lasagna pan with foil, then pour ½ cup water or chicken broth (enough to coat the foil with a millimeter or so of liquid). Cover with foil and place in oven.

2.  Heat up a large sauce pan over medium high heat on stove. Spray with cooking spray or oil of choice. In batches, sear meatballs on all sides over a period of 5 minutes. Pull back foil from oven pan, transfer meatballs and re-cover with foil. Finish baking in the oven for 10 minutes for each batch.

3.  Remove balls and serve! Balls should be firm, but not hard to touch.

## 12. Roasted Garlic Toasted Quinoa

Preparation Time - 20 minutes

**Ingredients**

- 1 garlic bulb

- ½ tsp olive oil

- 1 cup organic quinoa

- 2 cups vegetable broth or water

- 2 tbsp olive oil

**Instructions**

1. Pre-heat oven to 375 degrees F.

2. Peel the outer layers of the garlic skin off, leaving the cloves still attached and chop off the top of the bulb.

3. Place bulb in aluminum foil and drizzle ½ teaspoon olive oil over the exposed surface of the garlic, letting the oil sink down into the cloves. Wrap the garlic in the aluminum foil and roast in the oven for 40 minutes.

4. While garlic is roasting, toast the quinoa. Heat a sauté pan over medium-low heat. Place one cup of quinoa in pan and toast for 4 minutes until golden brown and smelling nutty. Make sure to stir constantly so it doesn't burn.

5. When the garlic is almost done, make the quinoa. Place toasted quinoa and 2 cups vegetable broth in a pan. Bring to a boil and then let simmer for 15 minutes or till liquid is absorbed.

6. Once garlic is done and slightly cool, press on the bottom of each clove to push it out of its paper. Add garlic and 2 tablespoons olive oil to a jar. Place immersion blender into the bottom of the jar and blend into a smooth paste.

7. Stir garlic mixture through the cooked quinoa. Serve!

# 13. Zucchini Noodles with Italian Dressing

Preparation time - 20 minutes

## Ingredients

- 3 tbsp extra virgin olive oil

- 2 carrots (4 oz)

- 2 zucchini

- ⅓ tsp freshly ground black pepper

- ⅓ tsp garlic powder

- 1 tsp oregano

## Optional for dressing

- 3 tbsp apple cider vinegar

- ½ tsp spice

## Instructions

Noodles

1. Slice your zucchini and carrots and mix with the pepper, garlic powder, olive oil, and oregano in a pan. If a slicer is not available, you can get a vegetable shredder to achieve thin, long ribbons.

Dressing

2. Stir the apple cider vinegar, and spice (optional) together.

Salad

3. Mix the salad dressing with the carrot noodles and zucchini.

4. Keep the mixture in the fridge for 24 hours or serve at once.

# 14. Coconut, Cilantro and Lime Rice

Preparationtime - 20 minutes

## Ingredients

- 1 cup white jasmine rice

- 2 cups full-fat coconut milk

- 3 tbsp lime juice

- ½ cup packed cilantro, roughly chopped

- salt to taste

## Instructions

Stove-Top Coconut Cilantro Lime Rice

1.  Wash rice through running water a few times.

2.  Place rice, salt, and coconut milk in a saucepan. Cover with a lid and allow to boil. Remove the lid and moderate heat to low heat, and let it simmer for 20 minutes or till desired doneness. 15 minutes rice will be more al dente and creamier.

3.  Stir in lime juice and cilantro. Enjoy!

Instant Pot Coconut Cilantro Lime Rice

1.  Wash rice through running water a few times. I used a nut milk bag.

2.  Place rice, salt, and coconut milk in Instant Pot. Close lid and make sure it is locked and valve is set to seal. Set to manual mode for 10 minutes. Let pressure release naturally for 10 minutes and then do a quick release for remaining pressure.

3.  Stir in lime juice and cilantro. Enjoy!

## 15. Avocado, Dill and Lemon Zoodles

Preparation time - 10 minutes

### Ingredients

- 3 average-sized zucchini

- ⅓ cup of chopped dill

- 2 lemons, juiced

- 3 tsp. of olive oil

- 1 big avocado

### Instructions

1. Combine avocado, lemon juice and olive oil in a processor and blend until its smooth enough.

2. Wash the zucchinis, peel and spiralize.

3. In a big basin, mix zoodles, dill, and avocado sauce together.

4. Serve.

# 16. Shrimp Salad with Hot Bacon

Preparation time - 20 minutes

## Ingredients

- 2 oz chopped bacon

- 6 oz fresh spinach

- 1 lb. peeled shrimp

- ¼ cup apple cider vinegar

- ⅔ cup olive oil

- 2 chopped boiled eggs

Optional

- shredded cheese

## Instructions

1. Wash spinach, dry the leaves and divide between plates.

2. Fry chopped bacon on high heat.

3. Divide bacon and egg among spinach filled plates.

4. Remove moisture from shrimp. Pour olive oil in a pan, add shrimp and fry for 5 minutes.

5. Divide shrimp among the plates and (optional) sprinkle cheese.

6. In another saucepan, heat the bacon fat, and sprinkle the vinegar.

7. Pour the hot bacon fat over the salad plates.

# DINNER

## 17. Roasted Carrots with Ghee

Preparation time - 30 minutes

**Ingredients**

- 1 bunch rainbow carrots

- 1 - 2 tbsp cooking fat (ghee or coconut oil)

- salt and pepper to taste

**Instructions**

1. Pre-heat the grill to 400° F.

2. Line a baking sheet with parchment paper.

3. Place your carrots on the baking sheet in a single layer.

4. Brush the cooking fat over the carrots evenly.

5. Season with salt and pepper.

6. Bake in the oven for 20-25 minutes depending on desired crispiness (I love when mine start to brown on the top).

7. Remove from the oven and serve as a side dish or let cool and place in a container as part of your meal preparation for the week.

8. Enjoy!

# 18. Peppered Candied Bacon and Asparagus

Preparation time - 30 minutes

## Ingredients

- 4 – 5 pieces of uncured nitrate-free peppered bacon (keep 1 – 2 tbsp of the rendered bacon fat for cooking)

- 1 tbsp or more of coconut sugar

- 1 bunch of large asparagus (about 15 - 20 spears)

- 1 shallot, sliced

- black pepper and salt to taste

Optional
- 1 tsp or more of lemon juice (optional but brings out the flavors!)
- pinch of sea salt to taste

## Instructions

1. Preheat oven to 400° F. Line a baking pan with foil.

2. Place 4 - 5 pieces of uncured smoked or regular peppered bacon on baking tray.

3. Sprinkle with ½ - ¾ tbsp of coconut sugar. Make sure it's evenly distributed on bacon.

4. Bake on bottom rack for 15 - 18 minutes.

5. Remove from oven. The longer it cooks in the oven, the crispier. You can easily do this using a microwave if you need it done quickly.

6. Spoon 1 – 2 tbsp of the bacon juice into a bowl. Let it sit for later use.

7.  Once bacon is somewhat cooled, chop it into small pieces. Set aside.

8.  Next, clean your asparagus and trim bottom stems.

9.  Slice your shallot lengthwise.

10. Place the bacon fat in a large skillet on medium heat.

11. Add in your asparagus, shallot, pepper, sea salt, and a little more coconut sugar if desired.

12. Saute veggies for about 10 minutes or till asparagus is more golden and only slightly crispy on the ends.

13. Remove from heat.

14. Place asparagus on a serving dish and add your candied bacon bits.

15. Spoon any extra juice from the skillet over the asparagus/shallots/bacon.

16. Feel free to add more pepper/lemon juice/salt here if desired.

17. Enjoy!

# 19. Avocado Tuna Salad

Preparation time - 10 minutes

## Ingredients

- 1 avocado

- 1 can (5 oz) tuna

- 1 tbsp chopped red onion

- lemon juice

- salt and pepper (omit pepper for those on AIP diet)

## Instructions

1. Cut the avocado in half, remove the seed, and scoop out the flesh of both avocado halves into a bowl, leaving the avocado outer shell will a little flesh. (If on AIP, scoop out entire avocado flesh).

2. Add scooped avocado flesh, onion, and lemon juice to a bowl and mash together. Add tuna, salt and pepper, and mix to combine.

3. Fill avocado shells with tuna salad and serve.

# 20. Gluten-free Salmon Recipe

Preparation time - 20 minutes

## Ingredients

- 1 ½ lbs of fresh salmon, cut into 4 pieces

- juice of ½ large lemon (at least ¼ cup)

- 2 tsp Italian seasoning

- salt and pepper, to taste

## Instructions

1. Place salmon in a shallow pan and squeeze lemon juice over pieces. Make sure each piece is coated.

2. Let marinate in fridge for 1 hour (optional but if you have the time let it marinate).

3. Preheat oven to 500° F.

4. Place salmon pieces, skin side down on a parchment lined baking sheet or pan.

5. Cover each piece with Italian seasoning and sprinkle with salt and pepper.

6. Bake for 10 minutes.

7. Serve immediately.

# 21. Caprese Zoodle Salad

Preparation time - 10 minutes

**Ingredients**

- 2 zucchinis

- ½ lb heirloom cherry tomatoes

- 5 oz fresh mozzarella

- ¼ cup basil pesto

**Instructions**

1. Prepare your ingredients. Using your spiralizer, create your zucchini noodles. Cut the tomatoes in half. Cube the mozzarella.

2. Toss everything together and enjoy!

## 22. Watermelon Feta Salad with Mint

Preparation Time - 10 minutes

### Ingredients

- 1 watermelon

- ½ cup feta cheese

- handful of fresh mint leaves, chopped

- salt and pepper to taste

### Instructions

1. Cut the watermelon in half.

2. Using a melon ball scooper, scoop out the watermelon forming mini balls and set them in a separate bowl. Continue doing this until most of the flesh has been removed and the rind is hollowed out to resemble a bowl.

3. Sprinkle watermelon balls with feta cheese and chopped mint (reserving a little extra for garnish).

4. Toss with a pinch of salt and pepper.

5. Scoop the watermelon mixture into the hollowed out watermelon halves and top with any remaining feta cheese and mint.

6. Refrigerate for at least one hour or until ready to serve.

# 23. Marinara Meaty Eggs and Spaghetti Squash

Preparaton time - 25 minutes

## Ingredients

- 3 lb spaghetti squash

- 2 lb ground pork sausage

- 1 jar of classic Marinara sauce

- 3 large eggs

- 1 ½ cups of pitted green olives, sliced

Optional

- fresh basil for garnishing

## Instructions

1. Heat up oven to about 400° F, then bore little holes into a three-pound spaghetti squash using knife.

2. Set the spaghetti squash in a little bowl containing 1 ½ inches of water and cook for 25 minutes.

3. Let it cool for a few minutes, then cut the spaghetti squash wide open, remove the seeds, and slice the insides using a fork to from spaghetti-like pasta. Set to one side.

4. In a large pan, roast the ground pork sausage on medium heat and extract all excess grease.

5. Pour in the squash and green olives, and mix thoroughly.

6.  Add in your marinara and cook till the mixture starts bubbling. There might be need to continue mixing throughout the cooking to make sure the whole meal remains hot.

7.  When the mixture starts boiling, create a few divots and put three eggs on top.

8.  Seal the lid and allow the eggs to heat up, for 15 minutes. To achieve a completely cooked egg, the marinara combination must be hot all through.

9.  Serve with fresh, sliced basil and enjoy.

# 24. Chicken in Garlic Butter

Preparation time – 30 minutes

## Ingredients

- 3 lbs whole chicken

- ½ tsp ground black pepper

- 2 tsps sea salt

- 2 garlic cloves, minced

- 6 oz butter

## Instructions

1. Preheat oven to 390° F.

2. Season the whole chicken with salt and pepper.

3. Place the chicken on a baking dish.

4. Over medium heat, melt butter and garlic.

5. Drizzle the garlic butter over the chicken inside and out.

6. To marinate, sprinkle with the garlic butter in the baking dish every 20 minutes.

7. Bake for 1-1:30 minutes.

8. Serve with any side dish.

# DESSERTS

## 25. Healthy Homemade Cherry Gummy Bears

Preparation time – 30 minutes

### Ingredients

- 1 cup 100% tart cherry juice (I use Trader Joe's brand)

- 1 tbsp fresh lemon juice

- 3 tbsp all natural honey (or brown rice syrup)

- 3 tbsp unflavored gelatin

### Instructions

1. Combine liquids and honey in a non-stick saucepan and heat over medium-low heat.

2. Once mixture is hot, slowly whisk in the gelatin. Add about a ½ tbsp at a time so as not to create clumps, and whisk until gelatin is fully dissolved (the mixture should look glassy).

3. Place your candy molds on a cookie sheet and use a kitchen dropper/kitchen baster to fill the molds. Alternatively, you can pour the mixture into a measuring cup and pour it into the molds, but this may get messy.

4. Once filled, place in the freezer for 20 minutes.

5. Remove from molds and enjoy.

## 26. Dough with Pecan Toppings

Total time - 30 minutes

**Ingredients**

- ⅔ cup dough (a grain flour mixture kept in the refrigerator)

- 1 cup flour

- 1 ¾ tsp active dry yeast

- 2 tbsp sweet jam

- 2 large eggs

- ⅓ tsp salt to taste

- ⅓ tsp sugar to taste

Toppings (optional)

- 1 ½ cups of chopped pecans (about 8 oz)

- ⅓ cup of honey

- ¼ tsp of grated orange zest (optional)

**Instructions**

1. Heat saucepan containing dough over medium heat until it reads 115° F and set aside.

2. Combine eggs, the yeast, salt and sugar together. Add a little water and mix thoroughly until the egg mixture becomes very smooth. Add ½ cup of flour to the egg mixture and mix with a mixer. The whole process should take about 5 minutes.

3. Rub a clean bowl with oil or unsalted butter. Pour the remaining flour into the bowl and mix. Place dough in the bowl and coat the

dough with the flour/egg mixture. Cover bowl and set aside for 30 minutes for the dough to rise.

4.  Knead dough properly and allow to sit for about 15 minutes or until it swells up.

5.  Place dough in the oven to bake.

6.  Cool dough on a rack and then spread jam on it.


Described below is an alternative way to prepare the dough with the toppings.

Dough with Topping (optional)

1.  Set oven to 350° F. Place pecan nuts on baking sheet and cook for about 10 minutes or until they darken. Allow to cool for a few minutes.

2.  Place a saucepan containing a mixture of sugar, salt, orange zest, and honey. On low heat, simmer until a glaze is formed.

3.  Fetch a cup of glaze into another pan. Make sure you tilt the pan to allow the mixture to coat. Pour toasted pecans into the mixture and set aside.

4.  Spread the pecan toppings on the dough.

5.  Serve and enjoy.

# 27. Baked Buns

Preparation time – 20 minutes

## Ingredients

- ½ cup (1 stick) unsalted butter

- 2 eggs

- ½ tbsp dark brown sugar

- salt to taste

- ½ tsp ground cinnamon

- ½ tsp grated nutmeg

- 1 lb of dough

## Instructions

1. Beat mixture of butter, nutmeg, salt, sugar and cinnamon in an electric mixer set at medium speed until mixture is light.

2. On a lightly floured surface, form dough into rectangles of about a ¼-inch thick and 12 x 6 inches in size.

3. Get to the best position of work surface and spread the butter, nutmeg and cinnamon mixture on the dough with a 1-inch of dough border untouched.

4. Fold over the filling and roll the dough into buns. Pat sides of cut buns and rub to flatten. Alternatively, you can put a little flour on the edge and rub it smoothly.

5.  Transfer every piece of the buns into a saucepan and space out each evenly. Cover pan with a plastic wrap, and set aside in a warm place for about 45 minutes so buns can rise until they double in size.

6.  In oven pre-heated to 350° F with rack set at the middle, set the saucepan containing bun pieces. Before then, in a small bowl, make a mixture of egg and ½ teaspoon water. Brush bun top with egg and water mixture.

7.  Bake buns in the oven until they change color to a fine golden brown. Set a thermometer into the oven and when bun temperature reaches 185° F, let it cool. Sprinkle your choice of toppings over them and enjoy!

# 28. Buckwheat Banana Cake with Yogurt-Espresso Frosting

Preparation time - 30 minutes

**Ingredients**

Cake

- 1 cup whole wheat flour

- 2 cups buckwheat flour

- 2 tsp baking powder

- salt to taste

- 4 very ripe bananas

- 2 large eggs beaten

- vegetable oil spray (non-stick)

- dark brown sugar to taste

Frosting and assembly (optional)

- 4 oz cream cheese, room temperature

- ½ cup plain Greek yogurt

- ⅓ cup of powdered sugar

- ½ tsp espresso powder

- ½ tsp salt

**Instructions**

Cake

1.  Set oven to medium heat of about 350° F. Spray nonstick cooking oil on a 8½ x 4½-inch pan. Next, make linings of parchment paper with the longer side hanging over the side of the pan. In a clean bowl, make a mixture of buckwheat and wheat flour, baking soda, salt and baking powder.

2.  Mix brown sugar and banana in a separate bowl and mash together to get a creamy blend. Ensure all banana lumps are broken into pieces and sugar is entirely dissolved. Break eggs into the mixture and add some oil. Include all other dry ingredients to the mixture and stir together with a spatula.

3.  Transfer batter from the bowl into the ready-made pan. Ensure the surface of the pan is well coated with oil, then place in the oven. Bake until the cake becomes soft such that an inserted tester comes out clean without sticking to flour.

4.  Extract from oven and allow the pan to cool for about 15 minutes. Remove cake from pan and allow to cool.

5.  You could opt to bake cake and store it in an airtight container at room temperature. Cake can stay fresh for up to four days.

Frosting

6.  In a clean bowl, make a mixture of yogurt, salt, and cream cheese. Whisk the mixture together until well blended.

7.  Place a fine mesh over a clean bowl and sift sugar particles. Mix powdered sugar with yogurt and cream mixture.

8.  Stir resulting mixture in espresso powder. Spread mixture over the cake and serve.

# 29. Avocado Chocolate Mousse

Preparation time – 10 minutes

## Ingredients

- 3 pitted avocados

- ¼ cup of lime juice

- small white onion, finely chopped

- salt to taste

- small jalapeño (de-seeded if you prefer less heat), minced

- handful freshly chopped cilantro, keep some for garnishing

Optional

- ½ tsp of kosher salt

## Instructions

1. Mix the ingredients in a fairly large bowl: avocado, onion, jalapeno, lime juice, cilantro and a little salt.

2. Allow mixture to chunk. Run fork into the avocado mixture while slowly moving the bowl. After mixing, add a little kosher salt if you want, to your desired taste.

3. Use remaining cilantro to garnish, then serve.

# 30. Bowl Bread with Soup

Preparation time - 25 minutes

## Ingredients

- ¾ lb chuck roast, cut into cubes

- 1 loaf of bread

- 1 red bell pepper, chopped

- 1 onion, chopped

- ½ tbsp ground black pepper and salt

- 2 tbsp vegetable oil

- 3 cups of low-sodium beef broth

For garnishing (optional)

- 1 tbsp parsley (chopped), for garnish

- shredded cheese

## Instructions

1.  Make linings on a baking sheet using parchment paper. Allow your oven to heat up to about 340° F. Add a tablespoon of oil to a large pan. Fry meat cubes in oil and season with a mixture of salt and pepper. Cook and ensure you flip the sides of the steak cubes so that they are evenly cooked. After about 10 minutes of cooking, extract the steak and set to one side.

2.  Pour the remaining vegetable oil in the pan and add the bell pepper and onion. Cook for 4 minutes or until the onions are glowing and the peppers soft.

3.  Add beef broth and the steak to the onions and pepper in the pan. Mix properly and let it boil. Boil for 15 minutes so the broth can congeal and the flavors can meld.

4.  In the meantime, create a hole inside the bread by scooping the inside out. Set the bread on the baking sheet.

5.  When the soup is thick enough, spoon into the hole in the bread. Top with another slice of bread (which is not scooped) and cheese (optional). Place in pre-heated oven and heat until cheese melts with golden color.

6.  You can serve with parsley and enjoy.

# 31. Chocolate Hazelnut Mug Cakes

Preparation Time – 10 minutes

## Ingredients

- 1 cup chocolate hazelnut spread (about 10 ½ oz), divided in 2

- 2 large eggs

- ¼ cup of all-purpose flour (1 oz)

## Instructions

1. In a fairly large bowl, mix two large eggs with 8 oz (about ¾ cup) of chocolate hazelnut spread.

2. Mix resulting mixture with flour. Divide mixture evenly between two mugs.

3. Place the two mugs in the microwave and cook for two minutes each. Extract each mug from microwave and cool for five minutes each.

4. Use leftover chocolate hazelnut spread as sauce.

5. Serve and enjoy!

## 32. No-Bake Peanut Pretzel Granola Bars

Preparation time – 20 minutes

**Ingredients**

- ¾ cup peanut butter

- ¾ cup honey

- ¾ cup gluten-free pretzels, crushed

- 2 ½ cups oats

- 1 cup chocolate chips

**Instructions**

1. In a medium saucepan put the peanut butter and honey and place the pan on an average-low heat for 5 minutes or until mixed well.

2. Combine the remaining ingredients thoroughly in a big bowl.

3. Pour in the honey mixture and combine by stirring continuously.

4. Spread parchment paper on a deep dish pan and transfer the mixture into it.

5. Use another parchment paper to cover the top and press down the combination until it becomes firm.

6. Transfer the combination into the fridge for 2 hours or leave till it is ready.

7. Cut into bars and enjoy.

# SNACKS

## 33. Gluten-free Cranberry Pistachio

Preparation time - 15 minutes

### Ingredients

- ¾ cup cranberries (dried)

- ¾ cup pitted dates (soaked)

- ⅔ cup cashews

- ½ cup pistachios

- ¼ cup chocolate chips

- a little salt to taste

### Instructions

1. Set dates in the food processor and blend till they are cut into rice sizes. Include cranberries and blend altogether.

2. In a small bowl, add the cashews, pistachios and salt, and pound the combination into small nuts.

3. Include chocolate chips and continue pounding to reduce the size of the chips while the entire mixture bonds together. Add the date/cranberry blend to the pounded paste and mix thoroughly to form a dough.

4. Roll the dough into 12 balls and set them in the refrigerator for about 50 minutes.

5. Keep in the fridge and enjoy at any time.

# 34. Puppy Chow Recipe

Preparation Time - 25 minutes

## Ingredients

- 1 cup dark chocolate chips

- 1 cup creamy peanut butter

- 6 - 7 cups Rice Chex Cereal

- 1 - 2 cups powdered sugar

## Instructions

1. Melt peanut butter and chocolate chips together, either on the stovetop or in the microwave.

2. Next, add 3 cups of cereal to a large bowl. Pour one cup of your chocolate/peanut butter mixture over the cereal.

3. Add 3 more cups of cereal to the bowl and then pour the rest of the chocolate/peanut butter mixture on top.

4. Stir until the cereal is evenly coated. If there are pools of chocolate/peanut butter at the bottom of your bowl, add more cereal ¼ cup at a time until all that deliciousness is coating your cereal. Remember we WANT clumps, so do NOT add too much cereal!

5. Let the mixture cool slightly. I throw mine in the fridge or outside on my porch if it's cold there. You do not want it to harden!

6. Once your mixture is at or below room temperature, add one cup of powdered sugar. Mix until combined.

7. Let it cool for about 15 minutes.

8. Add more powdered sugar ¼ cup at a time until your cereal is coated to your satisfaction.

9. Store in an airtight container at room temperature.

# 35. Gluten-free Baked Eggs

Preparation time - 15 minutes

## Ingredients

- 3 oz of cooked ground beef

- 3 eggs

- 2 oz of shredded cheese

## Instructions

1. Preheat oven to 390° F.

2. Arrange beef in a baking dish.

3. Make a hole in the middle of the ground beef.

4. Crack in eggs and sprinkle shredded cheese.

5. Bake for 10 - 15 minutes.

6. Serve when it is cool.

## 36. Oven Baked Sweet Potato Fries

Preparation time – 20 minutes

### Ingredients

- 2 large sweet potatoes, cut into sticks

- 2 tbsp extra virgin olive oil

- 1 tsp powdered garlic

- pepper and salt to taste

### Instructions

1. Pre-heat your oven to 425° F.

2. Line a baking sheet with tin foil and place a cooling rack on top.

3. Place all ingredients in a large ziploc bag and toss to coat all the fries and spices in the olive oil.

4. Place the sweet potato fries on the cooling rack in a single layer.

5. Bake for 25 30 minutes, or until desired crispiness is reached.

6. Serve with your favorite dipping sauce.

# 37. Egg Roll Mozzarella Sticks

Preparation time - 30 minutes

**Ingredients**

- 5 sheets of egg roll wrappers

- 10 sticks of string cheese

- oil for frying

- marinara sauce

**Instructions**

1. Using a sharp knife, divide each egg roll wrapper into equal halves.

2. Take one of the sticks of cheese and a teaspoon of marinara sauce, and place them on one edge of the wrapper. From another end, fold the wrapper towards the edge with a stick.

3. Sprinkle little water on other edges of wrapper and roll lightly. Ensure that you press edge as you roll to ensure edges are sealed.

4. Repeat the process for remaining wrappers with the other sticks. Set cooker at medium heat and place a pan on it.

5. Pour a little oil in the pan and put rolls in it.

6. Fry sticks till they become light brown. Use a paper towel to drain excess oil.

7. Enjoy!

# 38. Pigs in Blankets

Preparation time – 25 minutes

## Ingredients

- 1 sheet of thawed puff pastry

- 6 hot dogs

- 6 slices of cheddar cheese

## Instructions

1. Set oven at medium-high heat of about 425°F.

2. Divide pastry puff into six rectangles of equal sizes. Put a hot dog on each slice of cheddar and place it on each rectangular pastry puff.

3. Roll and slice into three equal parts. Line a baking sheet with parchment and set three sliced pieces. Space pieces evenly with at least a gap of 1inch in between.

4. Bake until they turn light brown. Or bake for about 15 minutes.

5. Serve and enjoy!

## 39. Chicken Quesadilla

Preparation time – 10 minutes

### Ingredients

- 2 medium flour tortillas

- ½ cup chicken strips, cooked

- ½ cup bell pepper, diced

- 1 tbsp gluten-free taco seasoning

- black pepper to taste

- ¼ cup of shredded cheddar cheese

### Instructions

1. Place tortillas on a clean plate and microwave. When tortillas become a little crispy, extract from the microwave. Allow to cool; they will dry simultaneously.

2. Put the chicken in a clean bowl. Make a mixture of taco seasoning and pepper. Use the mixture to season chicken thoroughly.

3. Set cooker to medium heat. Heat chicken for 3 minutes, and peppers should have softened by then.

4. Spread cooked chicken over a tortilla. Spread cheese on top. Wrap dish with additional tortilla.

5. Transfer back to the cooker and heat for another 1 minute.

# 40. Bacon Sundried Tomato and Feta Rolls

Preparation time - 30 minutes

**Ingredients**

For Pastry

- 8 oz plain flour, including extra for dusting

- 6 oz of frozen butter

For filling

- 10 streaky bacon rashers, finely chopped and cooked

- 3 ½ oz finely chopped sundried tomato in oil

- 3 ½ oz feta cheese, crumbled

**Instructions**

1. Sieve flour and collect smooth particles in a clean bowl. Add a little salt and mix together. Use a grater to grate frozen butter into the mixture. Mix until butter is well-coated in flour.

2. Add a little amount of cold water (3 tbsp) into the mixture and mix to form a dough. Shape and make dough with your hand. Wrap and keep in the fridge for about half an hour.

3. Set oven to 390° F. Sprinkle a little flour over work surface. Divide pastry into twos. Put one part on the work surface and form rectangles of size 4 x 2 inches.

4. Put all filling ingredients across one edge of pastry. Use egg mixture (egg beaten with a little water) to brush other edge of the pastry and fold over the filling. Press pastry edges as you roll until a sausage is

formed. Brush sausage with eggs mixture again, slice into smaller rolls of length 1 ½ inches. Make 'V' marking on each sausage roll.

5.  Follow the same process for remaining filling and pastry. Line baking tray with parchment paper, set sausages on it and bake for about 20 minutes. Ensure the color of the sausage rolls is light or golden brown.

# TIPS AND HELPFUL HINTS FOR GLUTEN-FREE COOKING

**Be a master at identifying gluten-free foods.**

This may not be quite what you are expecting. And it's not a cooking tip either. However, anyone who wants to put a lifelong ban on gluten food items must understand how to read labels. You don't have to be a nutritionist to be able to do this. As a matter of fact, almost anyone can identify gluten foods if they could simply try to read the label of any purchased food item. This would give you an idea of which foods are safe to purchase and which foods are not.

Most times, people are just so unaware that almost every food item they purchase comes with a label showing the quality and nutrition of food. It's so unfortunate that many don't even care about the nutrition of items they purchase at the store. And this in itself has led to many uncalled for medical emergencies. It is not sufficient just to know that those food items like wheat and rye contain gluten. Many other food items that you cherish contain a heavy composition of gluten that you may not be aware of.

Learning to read labels carefully will do you lots of good in the war against gluten. It would also make you open to different food options.

**Have you tried chickpea flour?**

Have you tried out chickpea flour yet? If you haven't you are missing a lot. You could use chickpea for basically any type of cooking. It contains a high amount of protein and is a wonderful gluten-free cooking item you must have, as it is very affordable and multifunctional. Chickpea flour can be used to make different varieties of sauces, omelets, and tasty quiches. A solution of chickpea and water gives a crispy mixture close to beer batter.

## Explore a wide variety of grains

In layman's terms, gluten food items are mostly "grain food" such as rye, wheat and the rest. This has made many stick to rice as the only gluten-free grain out there. The truth is that there are more options of gluten-free grain foods out there but many people never get to try them out. Apart from rice and quinoa, other gluten-free grains include: tapioca, fava, amaranth, buckwheat, and teff. Each grain has its own uniqueness in taste and can be used as side dishes.

## Breadcrumbs, can you eat them?

Not all bread contain gluten. Some breadcrumbs are gluten-free and that does mean that you can consume them. Instead of purchasing, you can choose to prepare them yourself. Pulse excess home-made bread in a food processor and keep the crumbs in the freezer. Breadcrumbs are also important when you want to bake gluten-free meals but are not getting the results you desire. Gluten-free items that can serve as alternatives to breadcrumbs are cornmeal, quinoa flakes, and corn flakes or even rolled oats. These are great recipes that can provide a wide range of options for gluten-free cooking.

## Wraps! Don't take them completely out of the picture

Yes, tortillas may be completely out of the picture, but don't discard wraps yet. You can prepare tostadas, tacos and varieties of tamales. Or you could even choose to do away with the grains altogether and wrap your favorite meals in veggies like cabbage, Swiss chard and make delicious, healthy wraps. Just get creative about it!

## Don't throw away the flavor

For the sake of good health, many people stay away from gluten foods. However, due to the limited options and the need to rid their favorite meals of gluten, they end up watering down the flavor. Ridding food of gluten doesn't mean you must sacrifice flavor. If you consume gluten-free grains, for example, you may want to spice them up with condiments and spices such as; gluten-free tamari, varieties of sauces or veggie broth and Worcestershire (gluten-free) sauce. You can spice or top gluten-free foods with whatever you want. Only ensure your toppings are gluten-free whether they are homemade or purchased.

## Avoid white meat

It's hard to stop eating meat. No matter what health risks are involved. If you are on gluten-free regime however, totally stay away from "white meat" or "seitan". Seitan contains up to 80% of gluten if not more. This is a no go area for those on gluten-free menu. Alternatively, there are meatless alternatives that are healthier and gluten-free, tempeh and tofu being classic examples. Other alternatives to white meat include mushrooms, gluten-free cheesesteaks, and jackfruit.

With these options, you can make your own gluten-free white meat as substitute for the fresh variety.

## Read articles on gluten recipes

You would find a rich source of information on gluten-free recipes to digest on blogs, websites, online forms, etc. You would get to meet experts on forums and they can share a thing or two. The more you read and study, the more you understand gluten-free recipes, and how to substitute them when cooking to get desired results. Also, you'd learn how to create more varieties of your food and make other exciting discoveries yourself.

## Keep it simple

All you need to focus on are foods that are naturally gluten-free. And yes, there may be gluten-free versions of almost any kind of food, but that doesn't mean they are healthy enough. It is best to stick to naturally gluten-free foods than processed ones. It is best, if you can prepare these foods yourself using the cooking instructions provided already. Gluten-free foods may feel very inconvenient at the start, but as you get used to it, you will reap great dividends and they will naturally become second nature to you. Vegetables such as carrots, potatoes, and fruits are options to quench immediate hunger with instead of resorting to buying processed foods.

# TIPS TO SUCCESSFUL FOOD SHOPPING

The best tip for a successful food shopping campaign is having a shopping list. A shopping list is an organized, detailed list of food items or supplies that you need over a period of time. Successful food shopping is well planned and prepared for. Urgency is one thing, preparation is another. When you purchase food items in a hurry there is a high chance you would definitely purchase an item that isn't just worth it. Before you go shopping, prepare and plan effectively.

Keeping a food list will also reduce the chances of impulse buying and spending on items you basically don't need. And perhaps, the greatest benefit of keeping a shopping list is that it helps you stick to a budget. When you have a budget for certain food items you want to purchase at the grocery store, there is a high chance you will leave the store getting the right items you need. Keeping to a budget helps you achieve your shopping goals and reduces the chances of impulse buying.

If you do not wish to go grocery shopping too often, then you need to make a list of staples. Staples include items like; gluten-free flour, fruits, dried fruits, cans of soup, tuna fish, bags of vegetables, sauces, bottled juice, cereals, pasteurized products, dry milk, powdered milk, etc.

Sometimes, visiting the grocery store can become extremely boring especially as you get older and you have a thousand reasons for not going. Also, moving around a large store can be quite difficult. In these cases, what can you do?

1. Use motorized carts. Some big stores have motorized carts especially if you are going to be doing a big spend.

2. You may ask an employee to help you out.

3. Some big stores have resting sections where you can sit and relax for a while.

4. Shop during hours of the day when stores are not really busy.

5. Proper shopping requires lots of time and energy. Take a rest before hitting the grocery store, take your time and purchase whatever it is that you want. Do you use the grocery delivery service?

If you opt to get your groceries online, you might want to check out the charges and other factors involved to see if this would help cut down stress. Many require you to create an online account to place orders and manage your shopping items.

## How to shop for healthy food items

Shopping for fresh and healthy foods could depend greatly on geographical factors. For instance, people who live in rural environments close to farms have better access to healthy foods than those who live far away. Many large farms and agricultural agencies are established in rural environments where there is much farmland for farming. Farmers who live in rural areas find it difficult to move around the city, so they simply set up small stores around their areas of residence. Most food items such as fruit and vegetables purchased from convenient grocery stores are not always in their best condition. This is because they would have been preserved with different chemicals and this in turn, reduces quality. How to maneuver this?

Get in touch with a rural grocery store owner. Tell them about your interest in getting healthy food items. Negotiate on how you can get their best items right to your doorstep. Strike a deal fair to both sides. If you are successful in this, you will discover most of your food items such as vegetables, fruits, and dairy products will be in the best condition possible.

## Shop for nutritious products

Some grocery stores have shelves with special labels that indicate food quality for you to identify healthy choices- e.g. sugar level, gluten concentration, fat concentration, etc. Always pay attention to these labels when you shop. Join a (CSA) community of supported agriculturists. Being a member allows some benefits such as buying very healthy foods directly from rural farmers at great prices. This can reduce your visits to convenience stores, as you receive a daily supply of very healthy food products on a regular basis. To join the CSA community or source for rural farmers in your area, simply visit the CSA website. The government has also intervened in the agricultural market through the Senior Farmers' Market Nutrition Program to make more healthy foods available and at very affordable prices. Remember that what you consume influences the overall health of your body.

Do all that it takes to ensure that you consume healthy, nutritious, freshly harvested foods. Farmers' association have made this possible, so joining any of these associations will do you lots of good.

# GLUTEN-FREE SHOPPING AND PANTRY LIST

Becoming a gluten-free person is never easy. Therefore, this grocery list is created to help you through the transition! Here we have generated a detailed list of gluten-free items you can stock in your pantry. You are now on your way to gluten freedom.

**Flours**

- Coconut flour

- Sorghum four

- Quinoa flour

- Tapioca flour

- Chickpea flour

- Potato flour

- Amaranth flour

- Almond flour

- Millet flour

- Brown rice flour

- Buckwheat flour

- Arrowroot flour

**Other dry ingredients:**

- Almond meal

- Chia seeds

- Cocoa powder

- Flaxseed meal

- GF oats

- Baking Yeast, Nutritional yeast


**Alcoholic drinks**

Good news! Experts and major celiac doctors have revealed that filtered alcohol are gluten-free because, the distillation procedure eliminates all gluten proteins from it. However, ensure that you review and confirm that the labels specify for barley (as seen mostly in beer and sometimes hard cider) because other forms contain gluten.

**Freezer**

- Gluten-free Pizza Crusts

- Berries

- Gluten-free hamburger

- Gluten-free bread

- Gluten-free hotdog rolls

- Gluten-free tortillas

**Other staples**

- Brown rice

- Wild rice

- Dried peas

- Dried seeds

- Tamari sauce

- Black rice

- Lentils

- Red rice

- Mung beans

- Soybeans

- Kidney beans

- Pinto beans

- Black beans

- Cannellini beans

- Vegetable broth

- Walnuts

- Pecans nuts

- Cashews nuts

- Macadamia nuts

- Almonds Nuts

- Cider vinegar

- Balsamic vinegar

- Bragg Apple Cider Vinegar

- Raisins, dates, dried cherries

- Vanilla

- Kosher and sea salts

- Spices

- Peppercorns

- Fresh and dried herbs

- Candied ginger

**Sweeteners**

- Organic maple syrup

- Cactus nectar

- Dairy fruit sweetener

- Brown rice syrup

- Organic cane sugar

- Sorghum syrup

- Pure fruit jams

- Molasses

- Applesauce

- Organic coconut palm sugar

- Chocolate chips (vegan)

**Baking ingredients**

- Potato Starch, tapioca Starch

- Cornstarch

- Xanthan gum

- Cornmeal

- Baking powder, baking soda

- Cream of Tartar

- Salt

- Cinnamon

- Nutmeg

- Ginger

- Cloves

- Vanilla

- Instant coffee (for baking only)

- Canned pumpkin

- Unsweetened applesauce

- Cocoa, chocolate chips

- Oil, shortening

- Rice milk or almond milk

## Condiments and seasonings

- Black pepper

- Garlic powder

- Italian seasonings

- Basil, onion powder

- Chili powder

- Caraway seed

- Ketchup

- BBQ sauce

- Gluten-free mayonnaise

- Tartar sauce

- Taco sauce

- Gluten-free Worcestershire sauce

- Peanut butter

- Jam

## Other fats

- Canola oil

- Coconut oil

- Grape seed oil

- Spectrum palm shortening

- Buttery spread

- Olive oil

- Vegan margarine

**List of items you should avoid while shopping**

There are a lot of delightful gluten-free choices available in stalls and shops: however there are some items that look enticing that you would like to pick but you should avoid. Some of them are:

- Barley malt extract

- Bulgur

- Farina

- Graham flour

- Semolina

- Oats (not indicated as gluten-free)

- Malt

- Syrup, extract

- Matzah/matzo

- Tabbouleh

- Noodles (ramen)

- Rye, spelt, triticale

- Bouillon cubes

- Teriyaki sauce (not indicated as gluten-free)

- Udon

- Durum

- Vegetable starch